Trick or Treat

A Halloween Costume Coloring Book for Kids

by Erica Basora

This Book Belongs To:

_____

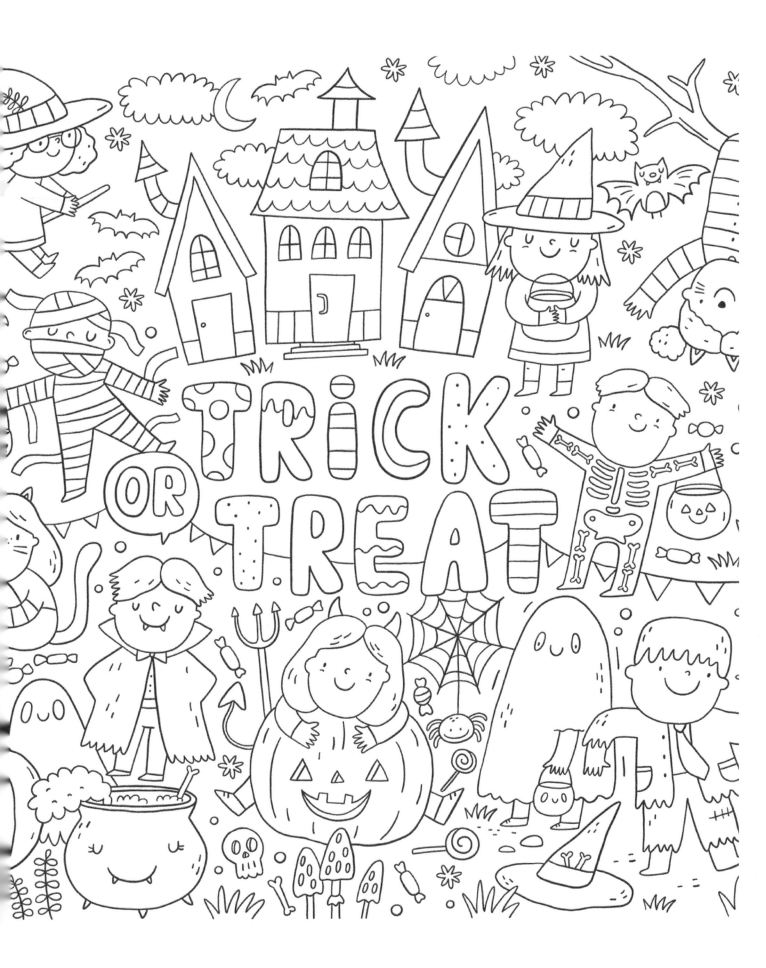

What costume will you wear this Halloween?

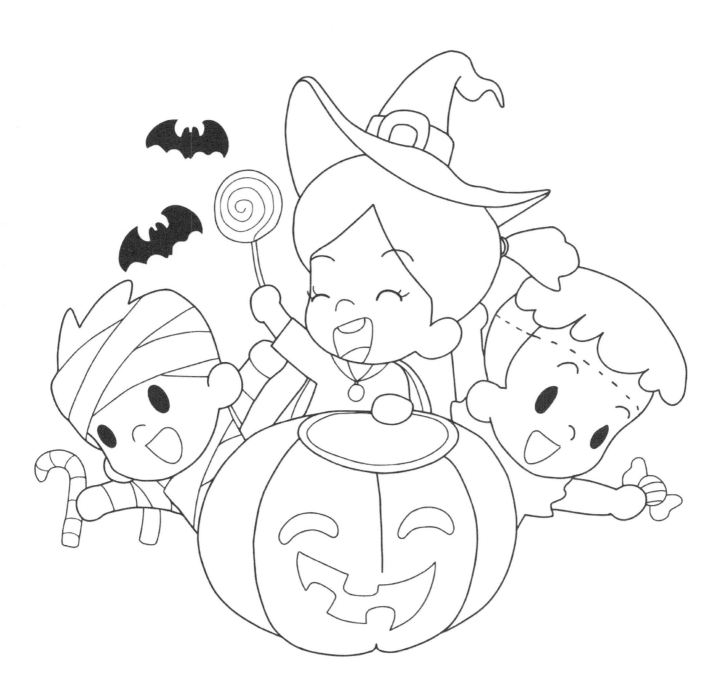

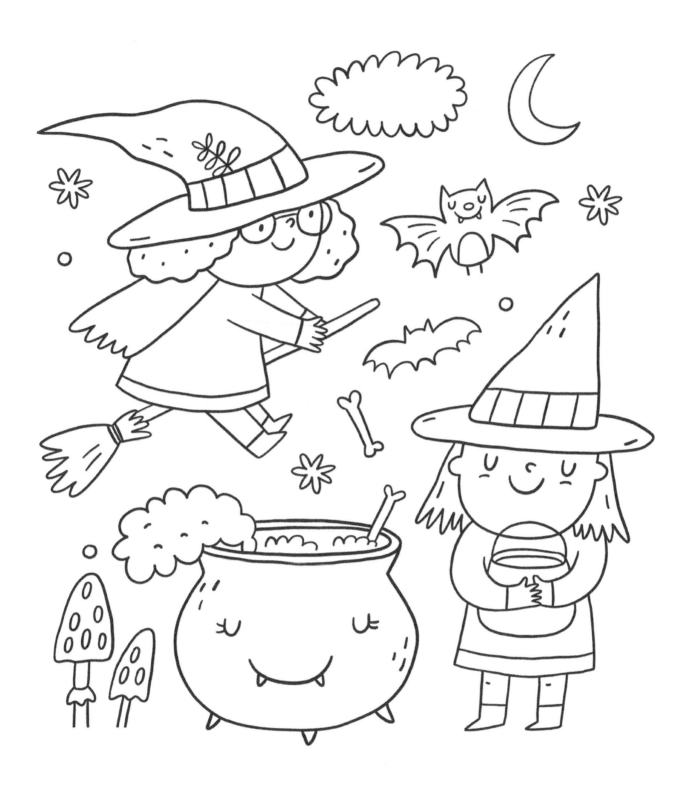

You can be a witch.

What Comes Next in this Candy Pattern?

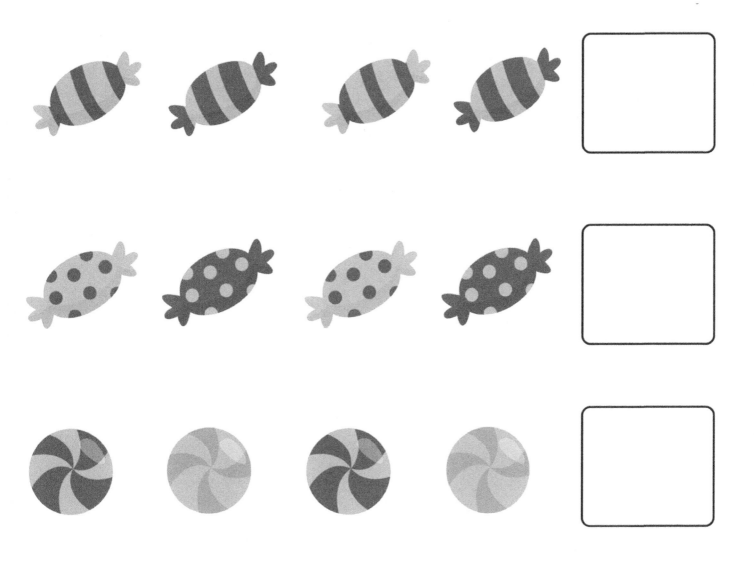

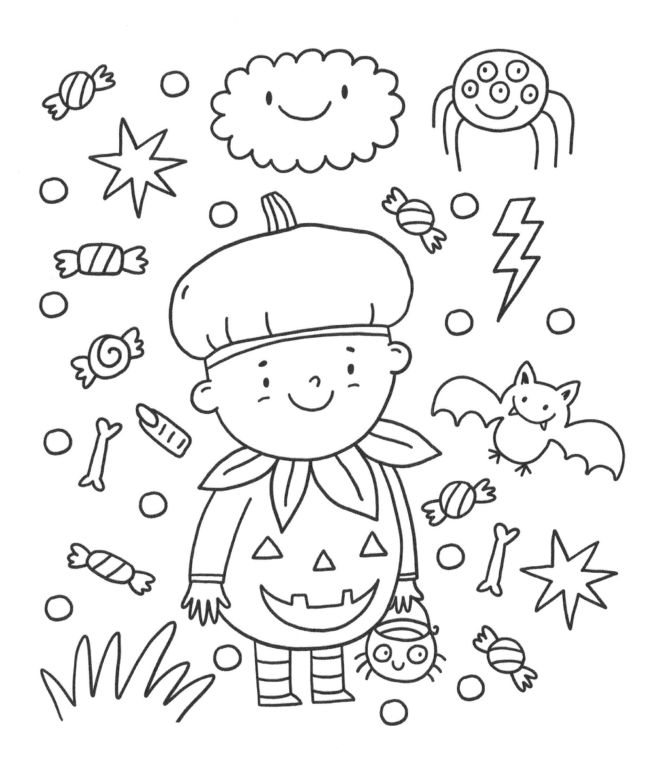

You can be a pumpkin.

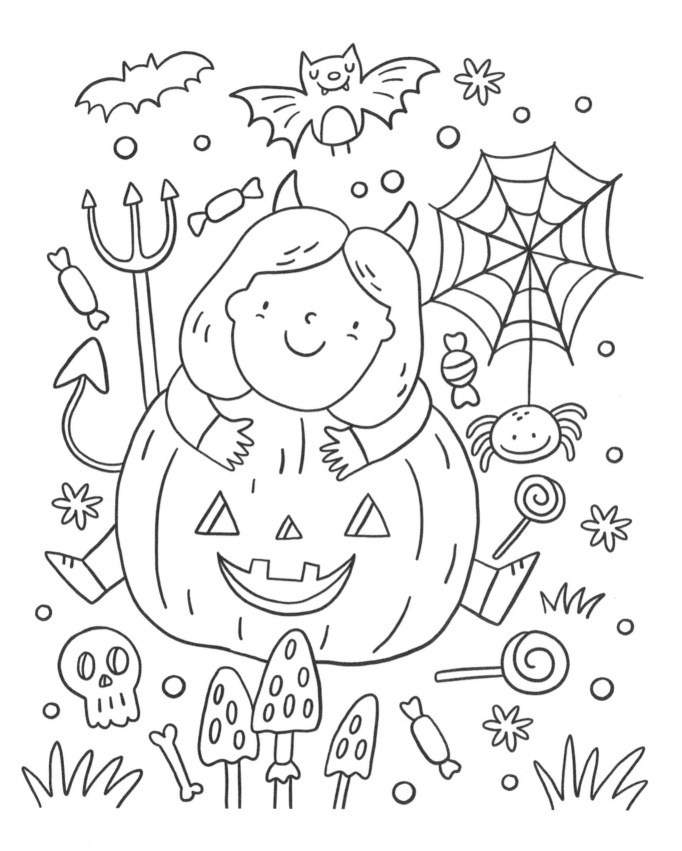

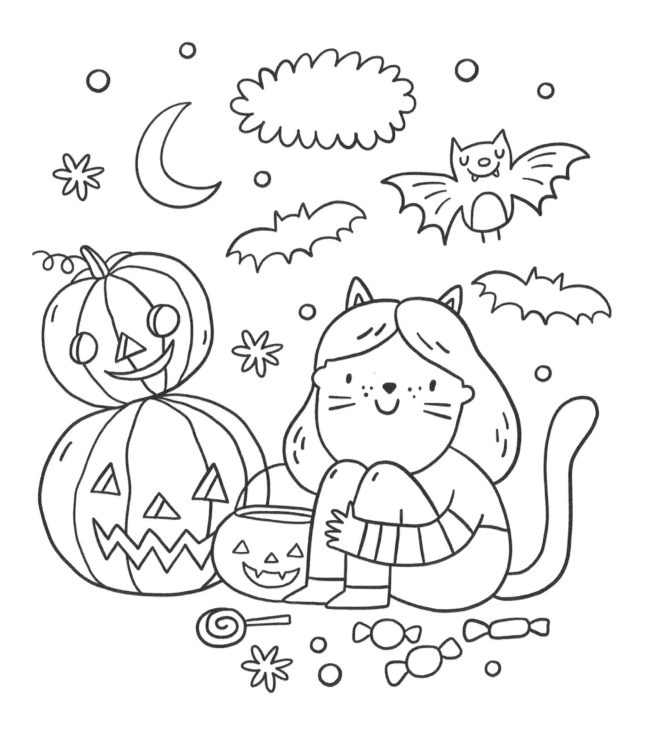

You can be a kitten.

Find the Matching Pairs

TRICK OR TREAT

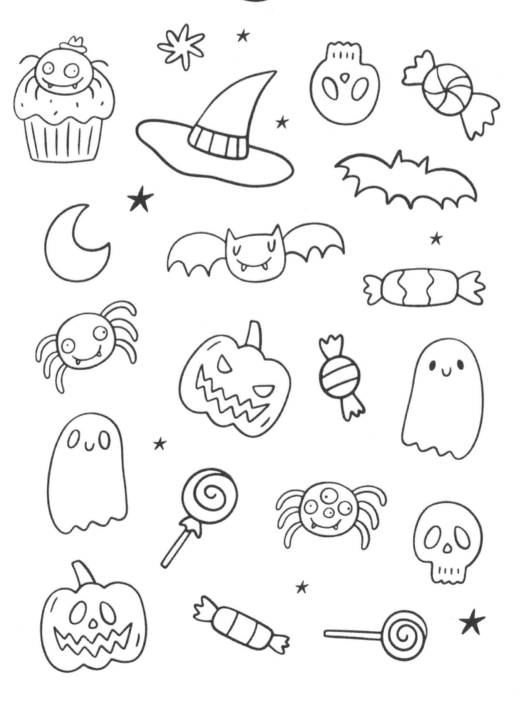

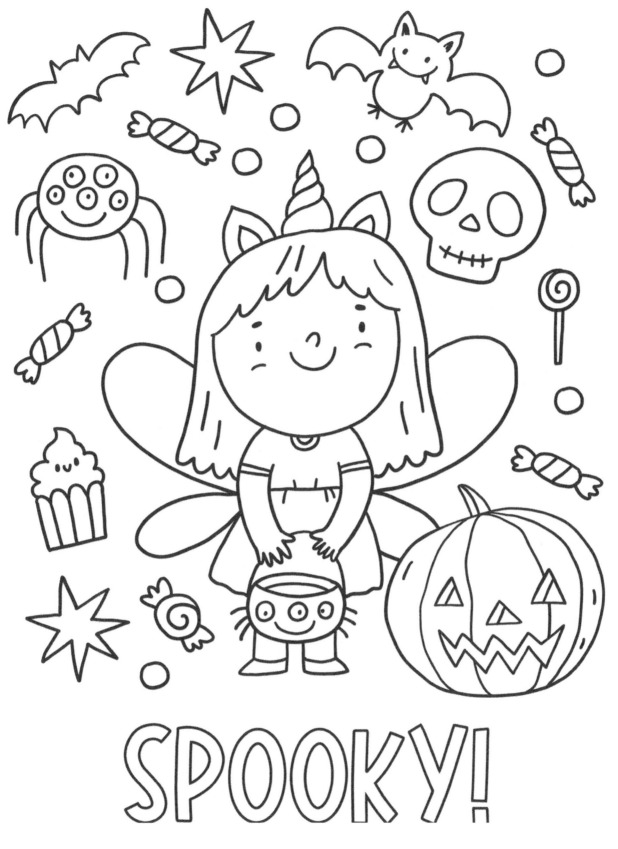

SPOOKY!

You can be a fairy.

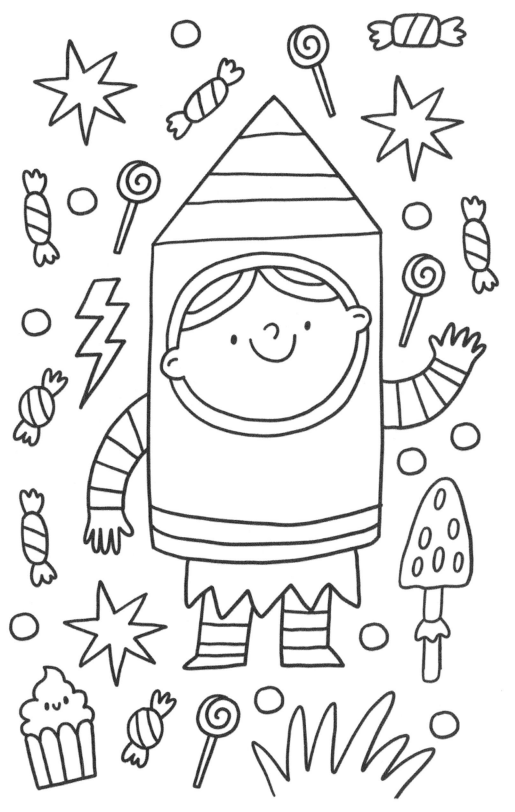

You can be a rocket.

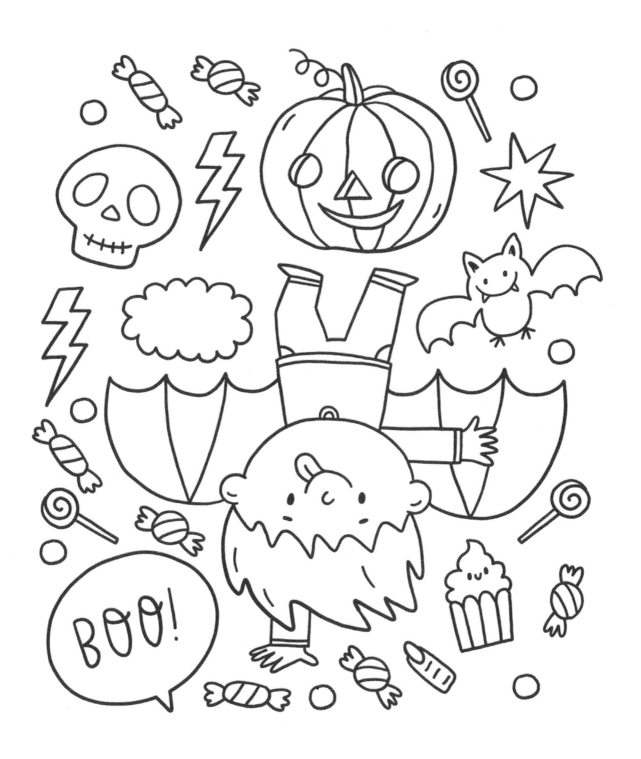

You can be a bat.

Trace the Lines

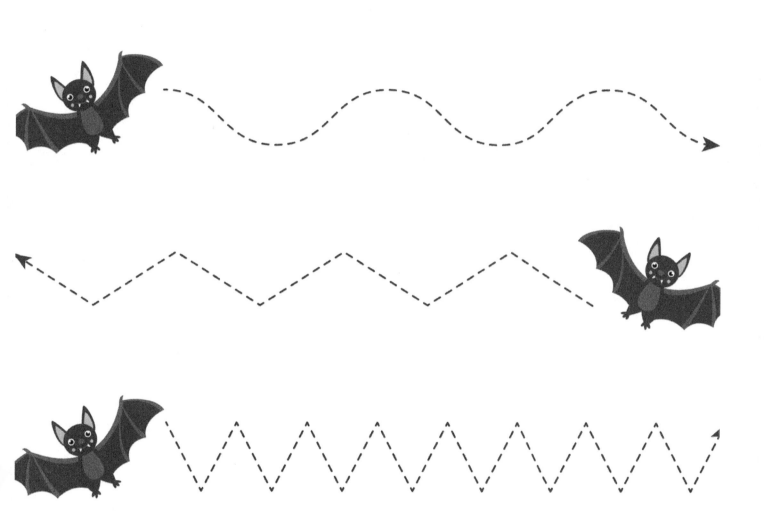

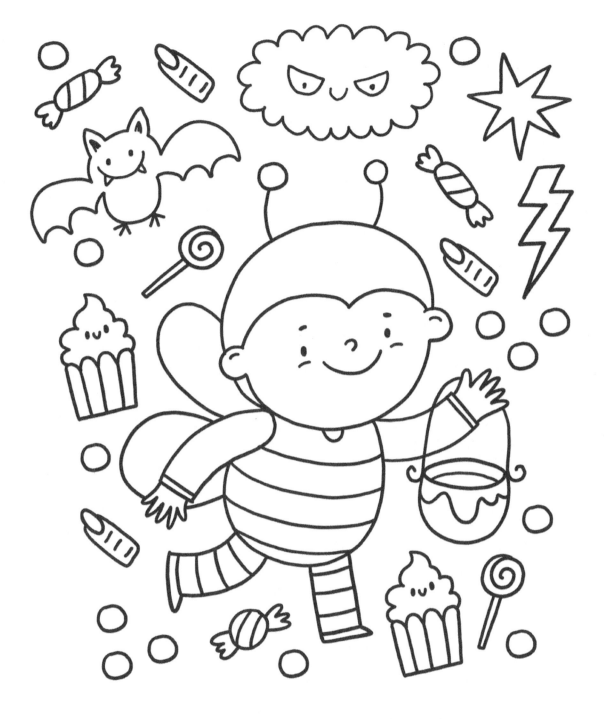

TRICK OR TREAT

You can be a bee.

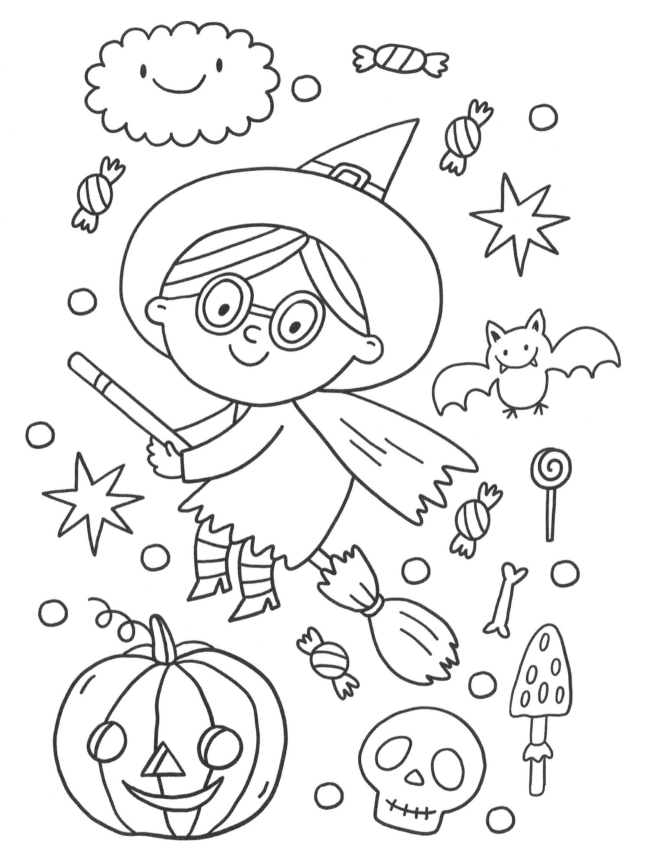

You can be a witch with a broomstick.

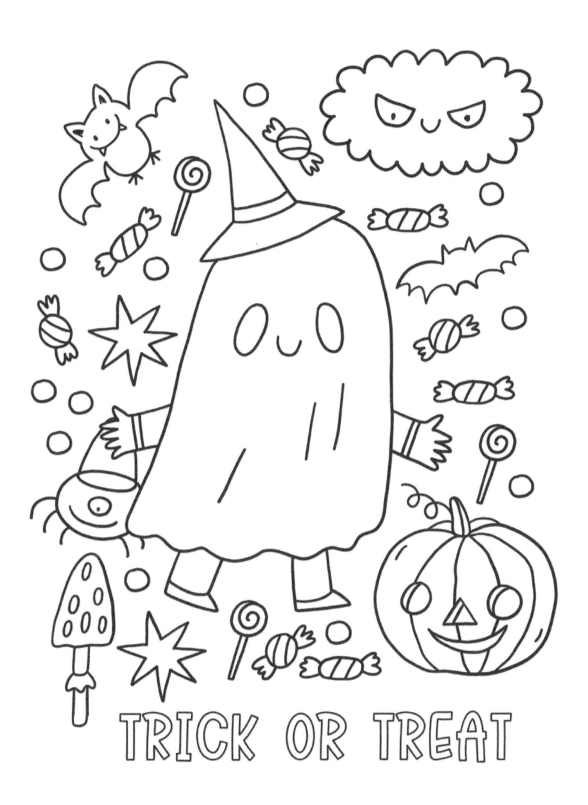

TRICK OR TREAT

You can be a ghost.

Maze game

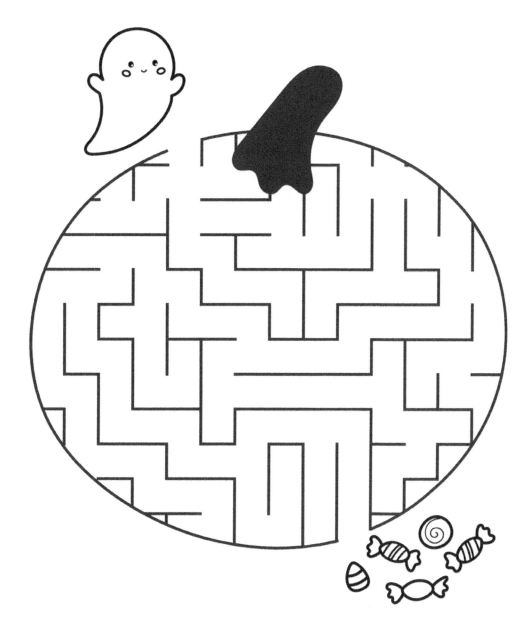

Help the ghost get to the treats.

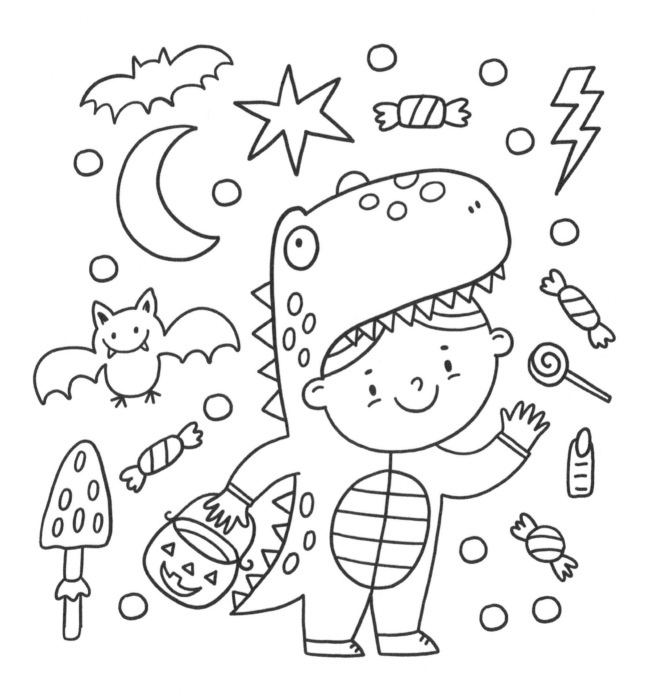

You can be a dinosaur.

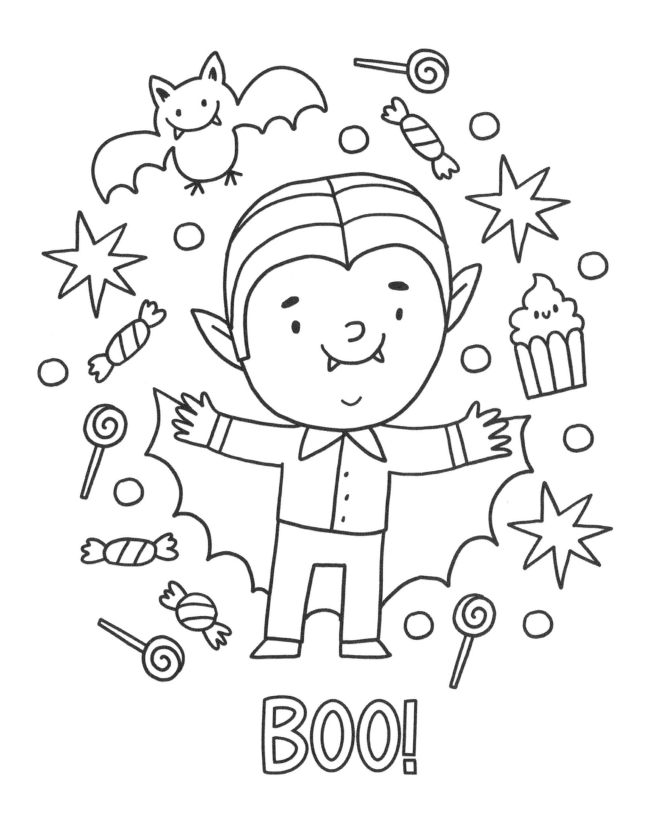

You can be a vampire.

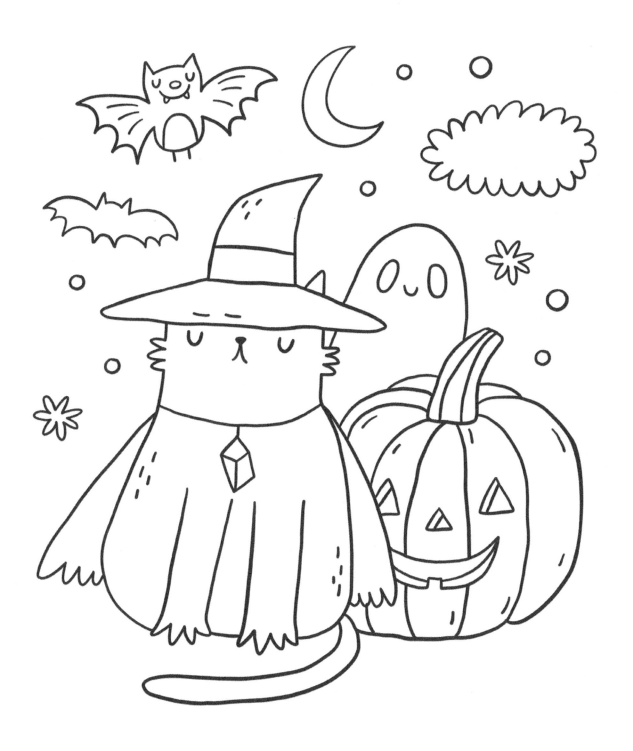

You can dress up your cat.

How many?

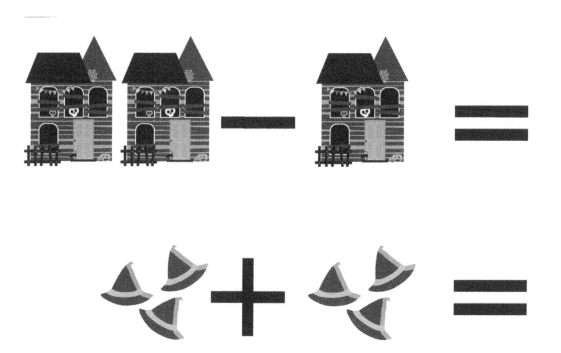

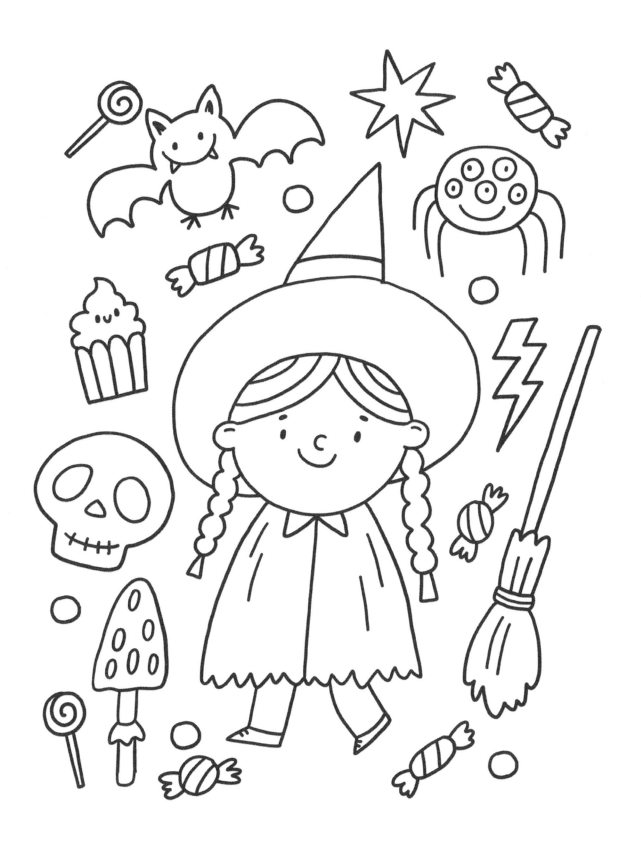

You can be a wizard.

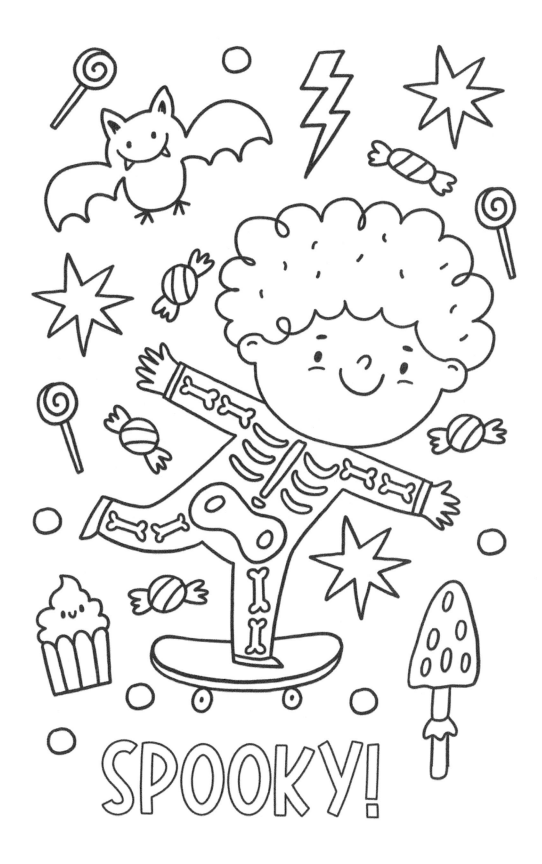

You can be a skeleton.

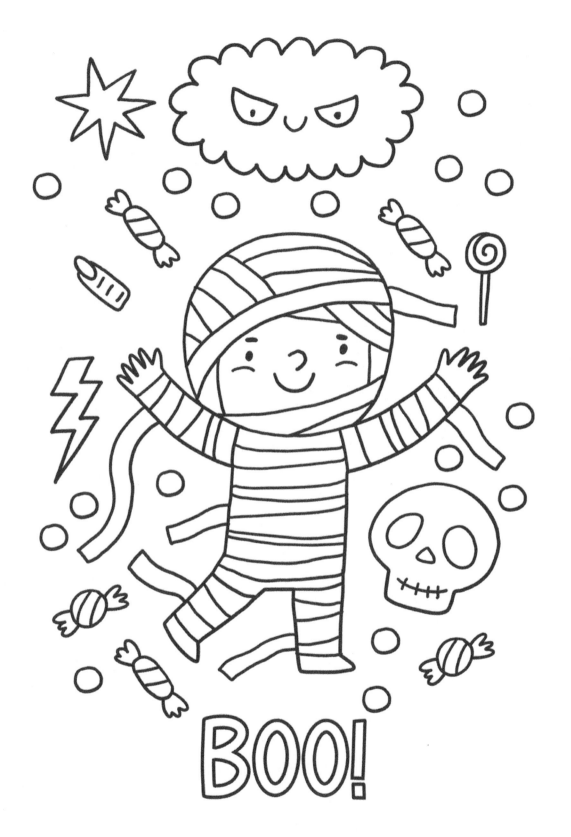

You can be a mummy.

Find the Match

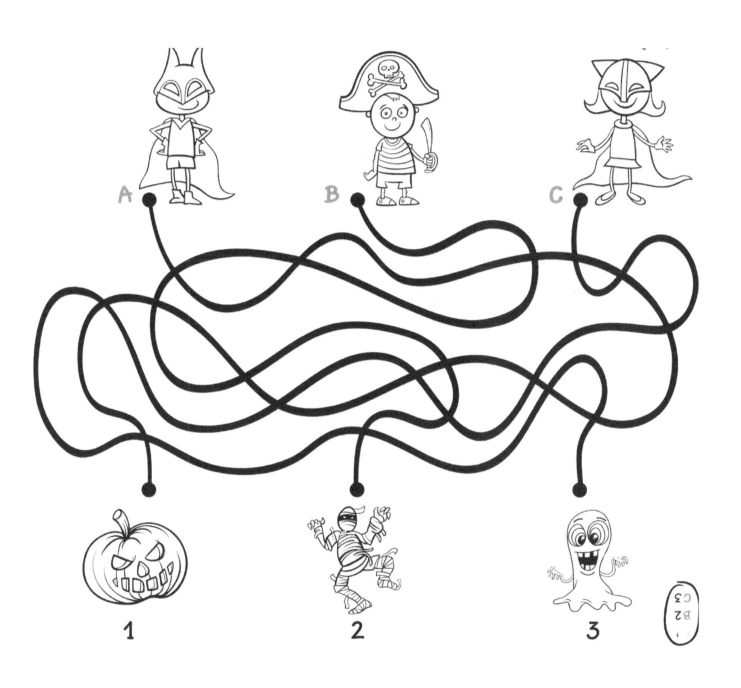

A

B

C

1

2

3

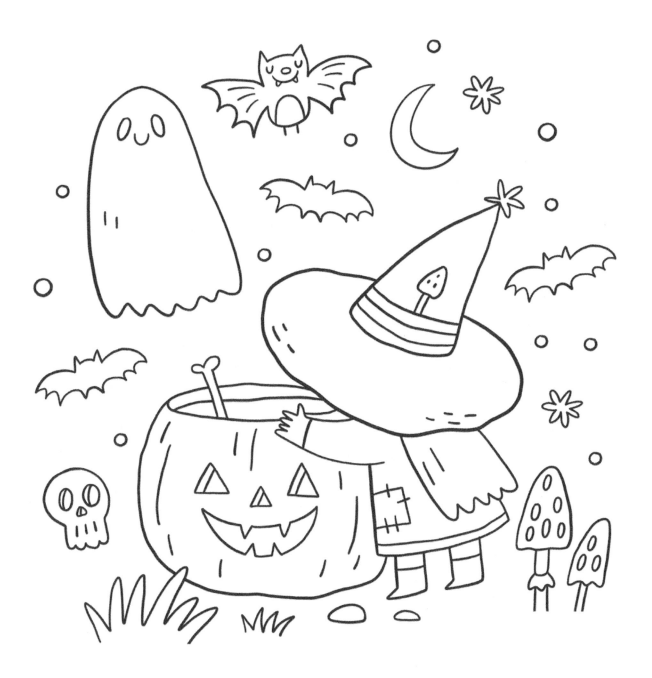

You can put on a pointy hat.

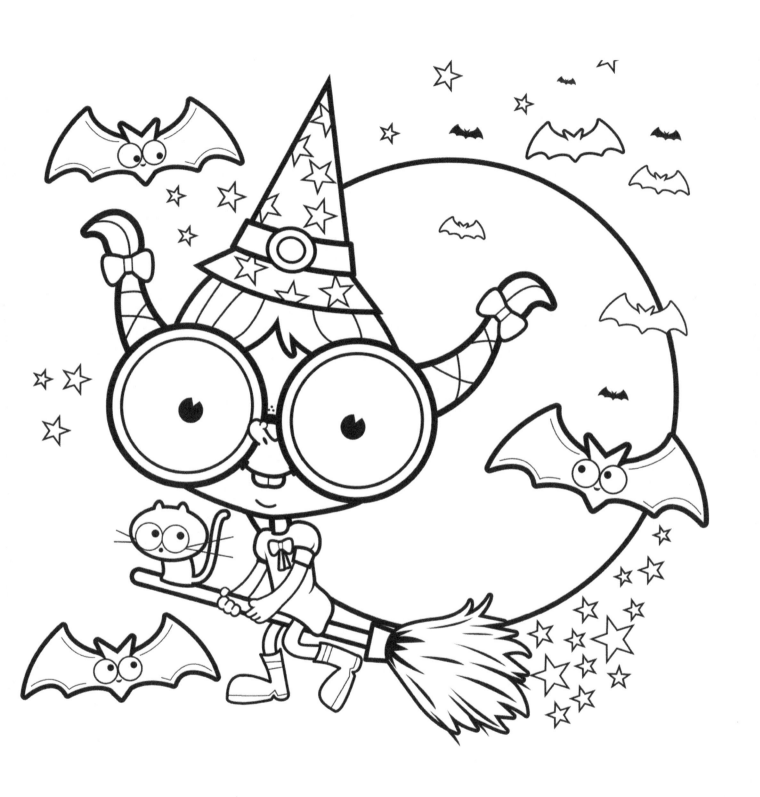

You can pretend to fly.

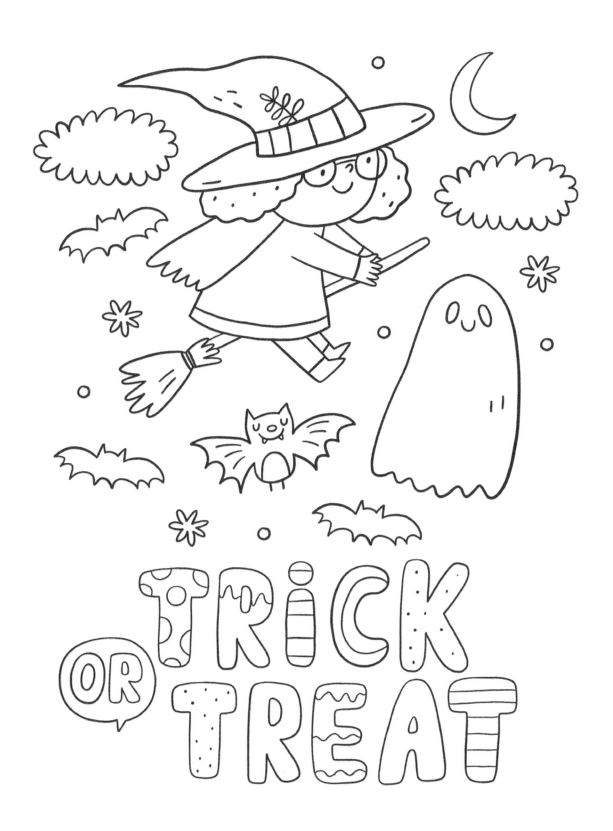

You can trick ot treat.

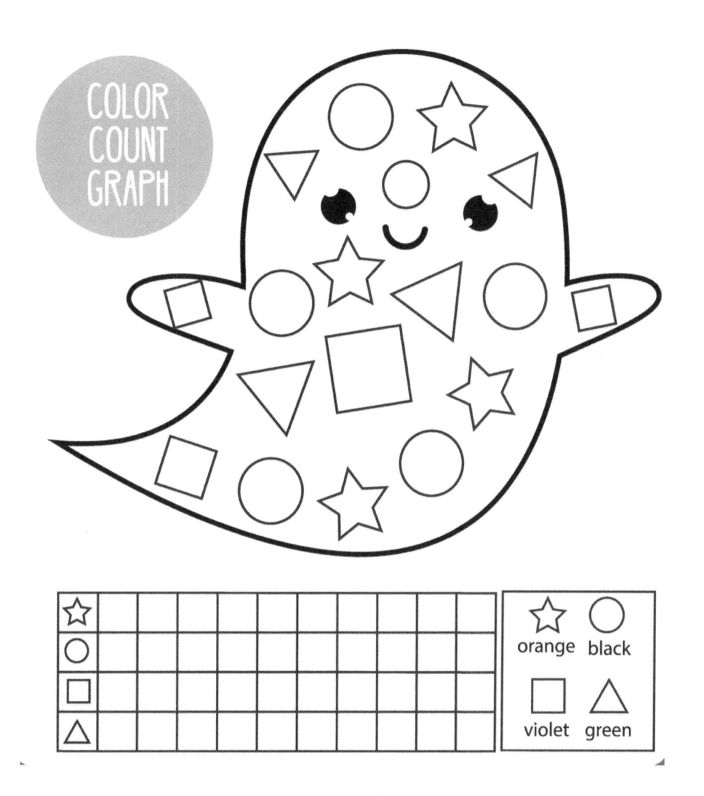

orange — star
black — circle
violet — square
green — triangle

Count the number of each shape in the ghost.
Color the graph with the number of shapes found.

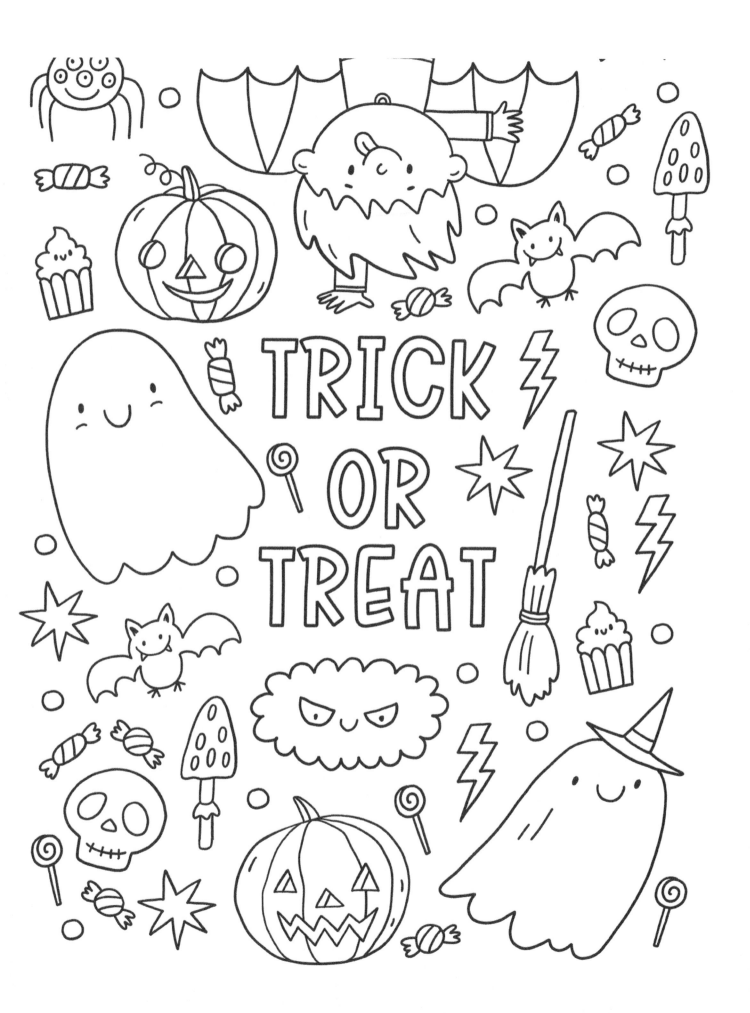

Made in the USA
Columbia, SC
05 October 2022

68749101R00037